AIDS
Acquired Immune Deficiency Syndrome

A NUTRITIONAL APPROACH

by
Louise Tenney, M.H.

The information contained in this book is in no way to be considered as prescription for any ailment. The prescription of any medication should be made by a duly licensed physician.

Published by
Woodland Books

Printed in U.S.A.

AIDS

Acquired Immune Deficiency Syndrome

A NUTRITIONAL APPROACH

by
Louise Tenney, M.H.

INTRODUCTION

There are more and more diseases inflicting mankind in this modern day and age. Viruses have been implicated in several scourges, such as Chronic Epstein-Barr Virus Syndrome (caused by a member of the herpes family), influenza, hepatitis, mononucleosis, and many other disorders. Infiltration by viruses have been linked to a breakdown in the immune system. The latest (and perhaps deadliest) plague, is AIDS. AIDS is an acronym for Acquired Immune Deficiency Syndrome. It is caused by a virus and is associated with a complete degeneration of the immune apparatus. Symptoms of this tragic disease are:
1. Swollen lymph glands which persist for more than six months
2. Fatigue
3. Fevers and night sweats
4. Weight loss
5. Diarrhea

Most viral diseases are highly contagious and can be transmitted through sneezing, coughing, etc. Until recently, it was believed that AIDS could only infect people via intimate sexual contact. However, the problem may be even graver than ever suspected. The September 28, 1985 issue of The British Medical Journal, Lancet, published a

1

study conducted at the Viral Oncology Unit at the Pasteur Institute, which revealed that the AIDS virus can still be virulent outside the body for as long as ten days. The AIDS virus has been isolated from plasma, serum, saliva, tears, semen, urine, cerebrospinal fluid, vaginal secretions and brain tissue. This certainly should concern every person. AIDS is not a disease which selectively chooses certain segments of society. The mainstream population should become aware and educated. JAMA 11/85 "A recent report from the Pasteur Institute in Paris...suggests that the AIDS virus might be pretty tough. The French study finds that the virus survives ten days at room temperature even when dried out in a petri dish." Dr. Richard Restak, a neurologist, states: "At this point, live AIDS virus has been isolated from blood, semen, serum, saliva, urine and now tears. If the virus exists in these fluids, the better part of wisdom dictates that we assume the possibility that it can also be transmitted by these routes. It seems reasonable, therefore, that AIDS victims should not donate blood or blood products, should not contribute to semen banks, should not donate tissues or organs to organ banks, should not work as dental or medical technicians, and should probably not be employed as food handlers." The problem is, the incubation period for AIDS symptoms to develop after a person has been infected can be a period of months to five years or more. How many people will be infected along the way?

CASE HISTORY

There have been many, many cases of hemophiliacs (people with a genetic blood-clotting disorder) contracting AIDS. This is a tragedy. Once infected with the AIDS virus, a person is infected for life. Hemophilia patients unknowingly can pass the virus to their spouse and unborn children. It is estimated that 90% of the hemophiliacs in this country have AIDS. There is a record on file of an entire family who came down with AIDS. The father was a hemophiliac and the wife became infected and it was passed on to the baby they were expecting. They had no idea at the time that the husband had the disease. The baby was born with respiratory problems, fever and an enlarged liver. He died a few months later. The family (including close relatives who did not have the virus) was ostracized, and treated like lepers by many people. Their story may seem unusual, but it isn't among hemphiliacs...innocent victims of the AIDS epidemic. (See McCall's, April, 1987 issue)

WHAT CAUSES AIDS?

HTLV-III (Human T-lymphotropic virus, type III) is considered the AIDS virus. There are two other viruses, the LAV, (Lymphadenopathy-associated virus), and ARV (AIDS-related virus) which are implicated, but they are all three suspected to be the same virus. The AIDS virus also goes by the name of HIV (or Human Immunodeficiency Virus). This potent virus attacks and destroys T-lymphocytes, the body's defense weapons against foreign and harmful agents. The T-cells are white blood cells. These white blood cells are divided into two subcategories, T-"helper" cells and T-"suppressor" cells. (Healthy people have a ratio of twice the helper cells as suppressor cells, or 2 to 1 ratio.) The AIDS virus avoids detection by other immune system "soldiers" by hiding inside the T-cells DNA. It attaches itself to the chromosomes of the cell, and replicates without opposition. The newly produced viruses then go on to attack other T-cells, until the body has virtually no defenses left. They also invade other body cells and organs until the entire system is infected. AIDS victims have a severely reduced number of T-cells. A question which has puzzled the scientific medical community is: Which came first, the chicken or the egg? Does the virus attack a healthy person and depress the immune system to the point of being vulnerable to other "opportunistic infections"? Or, because the immune system is already weakened, does the virus then obtain a hold and do its destructive work? Dr. Jay Levy, an AIDS researcher at the University of California, at San Francisco, believes that the immune system must first be altered. The immune system can be lowered through use of drugs, poor nutrition, stress, lack of sleep, etc. "If the person's immune system is not compromised by such events, I believe they will be able to fight off the virus and not develop the disease," he states. Persons who become prey to the vicious virus are then vulnerable to many other diseases. Homosexuals who have AIDS often come down with "opportunistic infections". They are called opportunistic because the depressed immune system allows the other bacteria the 'opportunity' to invade the body and cause problems. Dr. Alan Cantwell, Jr. M.D., states: "Most people with AIDS do not die from the pathogenic effects of one specific agent. They succumb from the combined damaging effects of multiple infectious disease agents..." The most common are:

PNEUMOCYSTIS CARINII PNEUMONIA: This is an infection involving parasites in the lungs.

KAPOSI'S SARCOMA: This is a cancer-like skin disorder involving tumors of the skin, lungs, lumph nodes, liver, stomach, spleen and intestines.

CANDIDIASIS: Candidiasis is a fungal infection which sets up residence throughout the body, and is manifest by white patches in the mouth and on the tongue.

CYTOMEGALOVIRUS: It is a viral agent which can cause blindness and other irreversible damages.

HERPES SIMPLEX: This is a virus that causes severe ulcers on different parts of the body.

HERPES ZOSTER: This is a virus which causes large blisters and scabs.

CRYPTOSPORIDIOSIS: Cryptosporidiosis is an infection caused by a protozoan in the intestines. It causes severe life-threatening cases of diarrhea. This intestinal disease is usually found in animals, but when involving AIDS patients, can lead to dehydration and malnutrition. There is no therapeutic approach (to date) which will alleviate cryptosporidiosis.

CRYPTOCOCCOSIS: This is a fungal infection which could lead to meningitis and severe central nervous system dysfunction.

A person may not know for a long time if he or she has AIDS. They may experience seemingly good health for many years, after contracting the AIDS virus. Meanwhile, the virus is insiduously infiltrating the eyes, brain, lungs, liver, spleen, kidneys and other organs of its victim. During this period of time the person may be virtually without symptoms. Carriers of the AIDS virus will be able to infect others by shedding the virus in bodily secretions. Once infected, the person will be infected for life.

When a person begins to show symptoms of AIDS, they are considered to be in "phase two" of the disease. Some health professionals have called this the AIDS related complex (ARC), or "pre-AIDS syndrome". However, by this time the person has AIDS, and probably has been harboring the virus for many years. The AIDS virus can invade the brain and cause a person to become demented.

The third phase of the disease is manifest when the immune system completely breaks down and paves the way for the "opportunistic infections". The person is completely vulnerable to any foreign agent-- be it bacterium, fungus, parasite or virus. There are also "auto-immune" diseases. They are called "AIDS-related diseases" due to the nature of the illness, being caused by viruses. The damaged immune system makes the person with these diseases more susceptible to infections such as AIDS. Auto-immune diseases are diseases in which the body literally attacks itself because it thinks it is a foreign substance. The body becomes allergic to itself and manifests this through inflammation, pain and other disorders. Some of these "auto-immune" and virus-caused diseases include:

GUILLAIN-BARRE SYNDROME: This disease of the immune system is characterized by progressive paralysis. It has been linked to innoculations, most specifically the "swine flu" vaccine of 1976.

EPSTEIN-BARR VIRUS: This virus produces extreme fatigue in its victims and causes mononucleosis and other debilitating infections.

MYASTHENIA GRAVIS: This is a chronic neuromuscular disease characterized by weakness and rapid fatigue of the voluntary muscles. The muscles around the eyes and in the throat are the most commonly affected.

SHINGLES (Herpes zoster): This disease is manifest by papules on the skin and severe pain. Shingles affect the nerve endings in the skin.

LUPUS: The technical name of this disease is "systemic lupus erythematosus". This auto-immune disorder is caused by antibodies in the blood attacking most of the tissues in the body. This causes widespread damage to the internal organs and is a very serious disease.

RHEUMATOID ARTHRITIS: It is suspected of being caused by the Epstein-Barr virus and causes general inflammation throughout the entire body. It involves the heart, blood vessels, tissues beneath the skin and creates scar-like formations in the lungs.

TUBERCULOSIS: This lung disease which used to be common and then diminished has increased greatly since the advent of the AIDS virus. This is an infectious wasting disease affecting various parts of the body, in which "tubercules" appear on body tissue. (Tubercules are small, rounded projections, swellings)

HEPATITIS B: this immunosuppressant disease is thought to be transmitted through bodily fluids. It is manifest by fever, weakness, drowsiness, headache, abdominal discomfort, and jaundice. Hepatitis literally means "inflammation of the liver".

5

HOW AIDS IS TRANSMITTED

Seventy-five percent of the people who get AIDS are homosexuals. Author Gene Antonio states: "During sodomy (anal-intercourse), the biological design of the rectum combined with the aggressive properties of sperm expedite their substantial entrance into the bloodstream. When this occurs repeatedly, antibodies to sperm develop, which circulate and impair the immune system. This happens both apart from and along with infection by the AIDS virus. It likely is a co-factor in HTLV-III infection". Any open sore or cut will allow entrance of the virus into the bloodstream. Intravenous drug abusers have contracted the disease through AIDS-contaminated needles. Bisexual males and prostitutes make up the segment of the population which spread AIDS. Even the most innocent portions of our society have fallen victim to AIDS. Hemophiliacs, who receive clotting factor concentrates made from blood collected in the U.S. are at risk for AIDS and many have become victims. According to the New England Journal of Medicine (and this was two years ago, in 1985), nine thousand hemophiliacs plus an additional twenty thousand other blood transfusion recipients have become infected with the AIDS virus. Homosexuals are discouraged from giving blood and a screening for AIDS is employed at blood collection centers. However, many donors may have AIDS without it being detected until it is too late. Dr. Roslyn Yomtovian stated in the February 7, 1986 New England Journal of Medicine: "There are now published case reports of individuals who are HTLV-III viral culture positive, but HTLV-III antibody negative. The frequency of such cases is currently unknown. Such persons may be unresponders to the specific inciting antigens or produce levels of antibody below the technical level of detectability...because data on HTLV-III test sensitivity are lacking or incomplete, all we can conclude is that the blood is now safer than it was before, but just how safe is unknown."

THE IMMUNE SYSTEM

A. Contributors to a Weakened Immune System

There are many factors which will contribute to an alteration in the human immune system. Among them are:

1. IMMUNOSUPPRESSIVE DRUGS: These drugs are given to cancer patients, organ donor recipients and others for medical reasons.
2. VIRUSES: Viruses cannot reproduce on their own. They take over the cells of the body and use them as virus factories. Some viruses mutate very rapidly and confuse the body's immune system, thereby infiltrating parts of the body where they usually are not able to go. They then damage cells, tissues, organs and break down the body's defenses even further.
3. STRESS: Constant, unrelieved stress will put a burden on the body, most specifically, the circulatory and nervous systems. It will contribute to the exhaustion of the adrenal glands, predisposing a person to hypoglycemia. The circulatory system will be affected and will manifest itself as high blood pressure; perhaps even heart attack or stroke. The nervous system trauma will show up as high anxiety, insomnia, irritability and lack of resistance to disease. Free radicals are formed in the body as a by-product of stress. Free radicals will attack the cells of the body, leaving them vulnerable to predation and suffocation by fungi, bacteria, viruses and other pathogens.
4. PARASITES: Bacteria are classified as plants, but parasites are considered members of the "animal kingdom". Parasites alter the immune system by neutralizing beneficial enzymes in the body and releasing their own toxic enzymes which kill white blood cells. They also release chemicals which paralyze the macrophages, and enter the body in such a way that it does not recognize them as foreign entities to be destroyed.

The parasites live off of the host (human) and deprive a person of essential nutrition, while distributing toxic substances throughout the body. It is believed by many that the AIDS virus is carried via parasites in bodily fluids. The parasites, and thence the virus, gain entry into the body through sores, tears or cuts in the skin or mucous membranes.
5. CHEMICALS: Many chemicals (which come in the forms of pesti-

7

cides, herbicides, industrial pollutants in the air and water, auto exhaust, cigarette smoke, food preservatives and additives, etc.) play havoc with the body's immune system by harming the DNA of the cells. The cells cannot fight the onslaught of toxicity and the liver (the detoxifying organ of the body) becomes weakened. The body responds with immune problems such as allergic reactions, or in the case of severe poisoning--diseases such as cancer.

6. CANDIDIASIS: This is caused by a yeast or 'fungal' overgrowth of Candida Albicans. Candida is a single-cell organism, and as it multiplies it develops toxins. These toxins spread throughout the body via the bloodstream and cause various chemical reactions. The Candida toxins send false messages to the glands and cause them to cease production of essential hormones. This creates confusion and the entire body is thrown out of balance. The fungus invades organs and produces a variety of serious complications.

Other factors contributing to a debilitated immune system are: lack of sleep, worry, depression, stress, antibiotics, alcohol, smoking, high-fat diet, faulty diet (white flour and white sugar products, junk foods), caffeine drinks, and foods fried in oil heated at high temperatures. Dr. Laurence E. Badgley, M.D. states, "It is probably no coincidence that in the U.S. and other countries, it is the urban centers which have the highest concentration of AIDS patients. Certain lifestyle factors within urban environments probably create large numbers of receptive persons who can easily become infected when exposed to the virus.

Every time a foreign substance enters the body, the immune system has to go to work. The U.S. food industry allows thousands of chemicals to be added to the things we eat and drink. The immune system is constantly on overdrive in the person who regularly eats processed, chemicalized foods. Most foods are grown with multiple pesticide applications, and undoubtedly carry a residue of these harmful chemicals. Indeed, a recent issue of Journal of the American Medical Association, featured a study which identifies a six-fold increase in risk of lymph tissue cancer among farmers who use certain chemicals on their crops. In the article, it is postulated that the chemicals suppress cell-mediated immunity and injure the thymus gland. Cell-mediated immunity is the type of immunity which is suppressed in HIV infected patients. In fact, the lymph tissue cancer noted in the farmers is one of the types of cancers seen in AIDS patients.

Another factor which probably contributes to immune system weakness relates to food preparation. Unlike other animals, the human herd cooks its food. Cooked food is laced with peroxidized fats, which induce free radical in the body, and cooked food is rendered relatively weak in vitamins, the free radical scavengers. Synthetic chemicals in water and air probably get their licks in this fray with the immune system. The virus is merely the K.O. punch.

B. Immune-System Strengtheners

Dr. Badgley has noticed that "a common trait noticed in AIDS patients is that those who take charge of their life do the best". An optimistic attitude does play an integral part in strengthening the immune system. The mind is a powerful instrument and can determine the course of a disease, in many instances. Herbs, supplements and a raw food diet can enhance one's immunity, and help stack the odds in the favor of health.

HERBS TO BUILD THE IMMUNE SYSTEM

Dr. Christopher's "anti-plague" formula is excellent for the immune system. The old-fashioned version of this preparation was known as "Four Thieves Vinegar". Richard Lucas in "Nature's Medicine's", published in 1966 relates the tale of the Four Thieves Vinegar: "In Marseilles, a garlic-vinegar preparation known as the Four Thieves was credited with protecting many of the people when a plague struck that city (1722). Some say that the preparation originated with four thieves who confessed that they used it with complete protection against the plague while they robbed the bodies of the dead. Others claim that a man named Richard Forthave developed and sold the preparation, and that the "medicine" was originally referred to as Forthave's. However, with the passing of time, his surname became corrupted to Four Thieves." (Lucas, 1966, p. 38)

Dr. Christopher's anti-plague formula consists of: garlic, apple cider vinegar, vegetable glycerine, honey, comfrey root, wormwood, lobelia, marshmallow root, oak bark, black walnut bark, mullein, skullcap, and uva-ursi. Because disease cannot flourish in a healthy body it is imperative that you keep your immune system functioning at its optimum level. This anti-plague formula has been used successfully by several AIDS sufferers in conjunction with a raw-food diet and various herbs and supplements. Disease germs are "scavengers" and can only thrive where there is an accumulation of toxins, parasites, mucous, etc.

GARLIC: This miraculous herb is one of the best that is known for eliminating disease. It is alterative, antibiotic, diaphoretic, diuretic, expectorant, antispasmodic, antiasthmatic, stimulant, antiseptic, disinfectant, tonic, nervine, germicide, and vermicide.

APPLE CIDER VINEGAR: The acid and other properties in apple cider vinegar kill many types of disease germs. The malic acid is similar to hydrochloric acid manufactured by the stomach for digestive purposes. It is an effective digestive aid. It helps maintain the balance between the acids and alkalis of the body chemestry. It is high in potassium for a healthy nervous system. Contains phosphorus, calcium, some iron, chorine, sodium, magnesium, sulphur, fluoride, and silicon.

GLYCERINE: It helps flush the cells clean of toxins and debris.

COMFREY: This herb helps promote the growth of strong cells and helps get rid of waste. It is rich in vitamins A and C. It is high in calcium, potassium, phosphorus, and protein. It contains iron, magnesium, sulphur, copper and zinc, as well as eighteen amino acids. It is a good source of the amino acid, hysine, usually lacking in diets that contain no animal products.

WORMWOOD: Alleviate pain, and gets rid of pin-worms and other parasites. It contains vitamin B-complex, and vitamin C. It also contains manganese, calcium, potassium, sodium and small amounts of cobalt and tin.

LOBELIA: Makes all the other herbs in the formula work more effectively. It is referred to as a "catalyst". It contains sulphur, iron, cobalt, selenium, sodium, and copper.

MARSHMALLOW: This amazing herb can help eliminate gangrene and peritonitis. It is an emollient which will aid in removing hardened deposits in the body. It contains 286,000 units of vitamin A per pound. It is very high in calcium, and marshmallow is extremely rich in zinc. It also contains iron, sodium, iodine, B-complex and pantothenic acid.

WHITE OAK BARK: This herb helps to tone and strengthen the entire system, including the cells. It contains vitamin B12, calcium, phosphorus, potassium, and iodine. It also contains sulphur, iron, sodium, cobalt and tin.

BLACK WALNUT: Black Walnut oxygenates the blood to kill parasites and fungus in the body. It is used to help balance sugar levels. It also is able to promote the burning of excessive toxins and fatty materials. Black Walnut is rich in vitamin B15 and manganese. It contains magnesium, silica, protein, calcium, phosphorus, iron and potassium.

MULLEIN: This herb has the ability to loosen mucus and move it out of the body. It is valuable for all lung problems because it nourishes as well as strengthens. The tea has been used for dropsy, sinusitis, and swollen joints. Mullein is high in iron, magnesium, potassium, and sulphur. it contains vitamins A, D, and B-complex.

SCULLCAP: This herb ennervates the nervous system, especially the spinal cord. It helps rebuild the nerves to good health. It is high in calcium, potassium, and magnesium. It also contains vitamins C, E, iron and zinc.

UVA URSI: This herb is useful for disorders of the urinary tract, also arthritis and cystitis. It should not be used during pregnancy in any large quantities because of the possibility of decreased circulation to the fetus.

OTHER HERBS FOR THE IMMUNE SYSTEM:

Many of the following herbs are called "sulphur herbs". They are beneficial to the immune system because they strengthen the tissues and purify the bloodstream.

BURDOCK: Burdock is one of the best blood purifiers. It can reduce swelling around joints and helps rid calcification deposits because it promotes kidney function. It contains a high amount of vitamin C and iron. It contains 12% protein, 70% carbohydrate, some vitamin A, P, and B-complex, vitamin E, PABA, and small amounts of sulphur, silicon, copper, iodine, and zinc.

CAPSICUM: This herb is also called "cayenne". It is useful when you want to rid your system of flus and colds. Capsicum is high in vitamins A, C, iron and calcium. It has vitamin G, magnesium, phosphorus, and sulphur. It has some B-complex, and is rich in potassium.

CATNIP: Catnip helps with fatigue and circulation. It alleviates aches, pains, nausea, and diarrhea associated with flu. It is high in vitamins A and C, and the B-complex. It contains magnesium, manganese, phosphorus, sodium, and has a trace of sulphur.

CHAPARRAL: Chaparral is known for its healing properties. It has the ability to cleanse deep into the muscles and tissue walls. It is a potent toner of the lymphatics and tissues. It is one of the best herbal antibiotics. It has been said that chaparral will rid the body of LSD residue. Chaparral is high in protein, potassium, and sodium. It also contains silicon, tin, aluminum, sulphur, chlorine, and barium.

ECHINACEA: Echinacea stimulates the immune response, increasing the body's ability to resist infections. It improves lymphatic drainage and helps purify the bloodstream. It is a natural antibiotic, without side effects. It has vitamins A, E, and C, iron, iodine, copper, sulphur, and potassium.

FENNEL: This herb helps balance the nervous system and moves waste material out of the body. It improves digestion and has diuretic properties. It is useful when there is cough and bronchitis due to mucus. Fennel contains potassium, sulphur, and sodium.

JUNIPER BERRIES: Juniper is an excellent disease preventative. It is high in natural insulin. It has the ability to heal the pancreas in cases of temporary damage. It is useful for infections. Juniper is high in vitamin C. It contains sulphur, copper, a high content of cobalt, and a trace of tin.

KELP: Kelp helps keep the glands healthy. It has a salubrious effect on many disorders of the body. It is called a sustainer to the nervous system and the brain, helping the brain to function normally. It is essential during pregnancy. Kelp contains nearly 30 minerals. They include iodine, calcium, sulphur, and silicon. It is rich in these as well as the B-complex vitamins.

PLANTAIN: Plantain will neutralize the stomach acids and normalize all stomach secretions. It has the ability to also neutralize poisons. It can clear the ears of mucus. Plantain is rich in vitamins C, K and T. It is rich in calcium, potassium, and sulphur. There is a high content of trace minerals in plantain.

PARSLEY: Parsley should be used as a disease preventative. It is very nutritious and increases resistance to infections and diseases. Parsley is high in vitamin B and potassium. It is said to contain a substance in which cancerous cells cannot multiply. It is rich in iron, chlorophyll, and vitamins A and C. Parsley increases iron content in the blood. It contains some sodium, copper, thiamine, and riboflavin. It also has some silicon, sulphur, calcium and cobalt.

OREGON GRAPE: Oregon Grape is well-known for the treatment of skin diseases due to toxins in the blood. It stimulates the action in the liver and is one of the best blood cleansers. It is a mild stimulant on the thyroid functions. Oregon Grape aids in the assimilation of nutrients, with its stimulating and purifying properties. It is a tonic for all the glands. It can be substituted for golden seal. Oregon Grape contains minerals such as manganese, silicon, sodium, copper, and zinc.

PEACH BARK: Peach contains curative powers. It strengthens the nervous system. It stimulates the flow of urine, has mild sedative properties and is useful for chronic bronchitis and chest complaints because of its expectorant properties.

PRICKLY ASH: Prickly Ash is a stimulant herb that increases the circulation throughout the body. It is beneficial in most cases of impaired circulation such as cold extremities, joint rheumatism and arthritis, lethargy, and wounds that are slow to heal. Prickly Ash is applied externally as a poultice to help dry up and heal wounds. Prickly Ash will help increase the flow of saliva and moisten the dry tongue, which often accompanies liver malfunctions, and is useful in paralysis of the tongue and mouth.

EPHEDRA(Brigham Tea): This herb is closely related to adrenaline and has some of the same properties. It stimulates the nervous system and acts directly on the muscle cells. It is used in the Soviet Union for treating rheumatism and syphilis. The juice of the berry has been given for respiratory problems. It contains substances that effect the blood vessels, especially the small arteries and capillaries. Its effect on the heart causes slower and stronger beat. It is considered a bronchial dilator and decongestant. It contains some vitamin B12, cobalt, strontium, nickel, and copper.

PAU D'ARCO: This herb also goes by the name "Taheebo". It is found in South America. It is used in some hospitals in South America. It is a powerful antibiotic with virus-killing properties. It is said to contain compounds which seem to attack the cause of disease. It is reported that one of its main actions is putting the body into a defensive posture, to give it the energy needed to defend itself and to help resist diseases. This herb contains a high amount of iron, which aids in the proper assimilation of nutrients and the elimination of wastes.

RED CLOVER: Red Clover is useful as a nerve tonic. It builds up the immune system by rejuvenating the liver. It is high in vitamin A

13

and iron. It also contains the B-complex, vitamins C, F, and P. It is valued for its high mineral content. It contains some selenium, cobalt, nickel, manganese, sodium, and tin. Rich in magnesium, calcium, and copper.

SARSAPARILLA: This valuable herb is used in glandular balance formulas. It increases circulation to rheumatic joints. It als stimulates breathing in congestion problems. Sarsaparilla contains vitamin B-complex, vitamins A, C, and D. It also has iron, manganese, sodium, silicon, sulphur, copper, zinc and iodine.

SHEPHERD'S PURSE: This herb acts as a stimulant and moderate tonic, especially of the urinary tract. It is rich in vitamin C. It also contains vitamins E and K. It has iron, magnesium, calcium, potassium, tin, zinc, sodium and sulphur.

STINGING NETTLE: In Europe it has been said that "the sting of the Nettle is but nothing compared to the pains that it heals". (LeLord Kordel's "Natural Folk Remedies"). The plant contains alkaloids that neutralize uric acid. It is rich in iron, silicon, and potassium. It is rich in vitamins E, F and P, calcium, sulphur, sodium, copper, manganese, chromium, and zinc. It also has vitamin D.

WATERCRESS: This herb can purify the blood and act as a tonic, supplying essential vitamins and minerals. The dried leaves are said to contain three times as much vitamin C as lettuce leaves. It is also very high in vitamins A, C and D. It is one of the best sources of vitamin E. It also has vitamins B and G. It is high in iron, iodine, copper, sulphur and manganese.

The sulphur-bearing herbs can protect the body from "free-radicals", which destroy the immune system. A free radical is a toxic chemical which is out of control, and which puts "holes" in cells and tissues.

OTHER HELPS

ACIDOPHILUS: This is the source of friendly bacteria. It helps the immune system fight harmful bacteria and fungus. It will speed recovery from antibiotics, which destroy the small intestinal flora responsible for proper digestion and B vitamin production. Biotin deficiency is improved with acidophilus.

CAPRYLIC ACID: This short chain fatty acid contains fungistatic and fungicidal properties. It is derived from coconut oil. It has been found to be very effective in killing off the candida strain of yeast infestation, without side effects.

EVENING PRIMROSE OIL: Evening Primrose Oil contains high amounts of PGE, a vitamin-like compound involved in proper function of the immune system. A shortage of PGE is believed to cause abnormal and harmful immune response. It stimulates the T-cells of the immune system. Experiments done in test tubes show that it reverts cancer cells back to normal cells. PGE is required for the T-cells of the immune system to protect the body from foreign cells, viruses, bacteria, fungi and allergens.

SULPHUR AMINO ACIDS

Sulphur-bearing amino acids are important constituents of the immune system framework. Through the sulphur they are able to make the mineral selenium available to the cells. We know that selenium is helpful in preventing cancer, and pulling heavy metals such as lead, mercury and cadmium from the body. They neutralize and eliminate potentially destructive free radicals which helps in cell immunity. The amino acids methionine, cysteine and taurine work as a team. During dieting methionine and cysteine will insure adequate taurine to protect the heart muscle from calcium and potassium loss.

METHIONINE: This amino acid helps keep hair, skin, nails and joints healthy. It functions to remove toxic wastes from the liver. Bottle-fed babies frequently have high ammonia content in their urine, which causes ammonia rashes and blisters. Methionine is the antidote.

CYSTEINE: This one is a powerful aid in protecting the body against radiation and pollution. It acts as an antioxidant, destroys free radicals and neutralizes toxins. It can block the chemicals in polluted air and tabacco smoke. It helps stop the toxic metals, mercury and cadmium from damaging sensitive tissue. Its antioxidant properties are enhanced when combined with vitamin E.

TAURINE: This is not an essential amino acid for most adults but is for infants. It is concentrated in the heart, skeletal, muscle and central nervous system. Taurine is associated with zinc in healthy eye function. It protects the loss of potassium in the heart muscle. It's synthe-

15

sis in humans is derived from the amino acids which play a vital role in aiding the immune system.

TRYPTOPHAN: This acid cleanses toxins from the blood stream.

GLYCINE: It helps in building antibody action.

L-LYSINE: This is one of the eight essential amino acids that the body must obtain from an outside source. It may lessen the incidence of some kinds of cancer. This amino acid can change one enzyme. It would appear that a single amino acid shift may underlie malignancy.

MINERALS FOR THE IMMUNE SYSTEM

CALCIUM: This element is healing to the body. It prevents heavy metals from accumulating in the body. Without adequate calcium the body absorbs heavy metals. It is destroyed by aspirin, coffee, stress, lack of exercise, lack of magnesium, lack of hydrochloric acid, mineral oil and oxalic acid.

CHROMIUM: Although only needed in small amounts by the body, this mineral is critical in fighting germs and foreign bodies.

IODINE: This mineral helps the thyroid gland produce the hormone thyroxine. It also helps the body absorb vitamin A. Lack of this nutrient can cause loss of interest in life and can promote a tendency toward obesity.

MAGNESIUM: When a person is deficient in this mineral they can experience a personality change. Magnesium produces properdin, a blood protein that fights invading viruses and bacteria. It is destroyed by alcohol, diuretics, white sugar, white flour, and a high-protein diet.

MANGANESE: It activates enzymes that work with vitamin C. As a team, they fight toxins and free radicals. It also stimulates the release of histamine, which protects the immune system. It is destroyed by high meat intake, excess phosphorus, and calcium.

SELENIUM: This is a very important trace mineral. It manifests anticancer effects. Cancer rates are lowest in regions with selenium-rich soil. It inhibits breast, skin, liver and colon cancer. Selenium is lost in food processing. Brown rice has fifteen times the senenium content of white rice. Whole wheat bread contains twice as much as white bread. Selenium and vitamin E work together to protect the body's cells.

ZINC: This mineral produces histamine, which dilates the capillaries so that blood, carrying immune-fighting white blood cells, can hurry to the scene of an infection.

VITAMINS FOR THE
IMMUNE SYSTEM

These vitamins have anti-oxidant qualities and help protect the immune system from free-radicals.

VITAMIN A: This vitamin increases resistance to infections. Deficiencies increase chances of viral, bacterial and protozoal invasions, and their severity. It is an essential nutrient to guard against cancer. Laboratory evidence shows that vitamin A is able to suppress chemically-induced tumors. This vitamin is involved with the maintenance of epithelial linings and mucous membranes, which are the first places that are penetrated by invaders. Vitamin A protects against the effects of various forms of pollution. The protection of vitamin A seems to be most evident among smokers. It reduces susceptibility to respiratory problems, i.e., colds, sinusitis, asthma, bronchitis, ear infections, and cystic fibrosis. It increases immunity against environmental pollution such as pesticides and herbicides. It works with zinc for optimum efficiency. Vitamin A is destroyed by high heat.

VITAMIN E: This vitamin prevents the oxidized state that cancer cells thrive in. It deactivates the free radicals that promote cellular damage leading to malignancy. Deficiencies of vitamin E depress general resistance to disease. Its blood-thinning properties help dissolve blood clots and keep the arteries from clogging. The antioxidant characteristics are useful in retarding the aging process. Bacteria, viruses, and cancer cells respond to larger amounts of vitamin E than recommended in RDA. Processing and storage of food destroys some of the vitamin E content of most foods.

VITAMIN C: This vitamin plays a role in the formation of connective tissue in the body. It also helps the body's absorption of iron. More importantly, however, vitamin C has shown even more powerful effects through animal, human and test-tube studies. It has been demonstrated that this vitamin can activate white blood cells to battle virus protein. Vitamin C has the ability to kill disease-inducing bacteria. Vitamin C can be affected by exposure to light, long-term storage of food, heat and canning.

17

B VITAMINS

B vitamins protect both the immune and nervous systems. They help build blood, protect the body against infection and help produce antibodies. They increase production of hydrochloric acid for digestion, and are very vital in helping stabilize mood swings. These are the vitamins that support the immune system by reducing the impact of stress in one's life.

B-1 (Thiamine): This B-complex vitamin is helpful for cell respiration, metabolism of carbohydrates, a healthy heart and proper growth of the body.

B-2 (Riboflavin): It is used by the body to metabolize proteins and lipids, supplies oxygen to the cells and is used by the skin and nails. It is especially needed during stressful situations.

B-3 (Niacin): This nutrient stimulates circulation. It aids memory function, releases histamines and helps in hyperactivity. It is an excellent vitamin for the nerves. It is essential for brain metabolism. It reduces tension, fatigue, depression and insomnia.

B-5 (Pantothenic Acid): It protects against respiratory infections and is a natural tranquilizer.

B-6 (Pyridoxine): The body uses B-6 in hormone and antibody production, in the synthesis of DNA and RNA and in the metabolism of fat, protein and carbohydrates. It is nature's diuretic and is very useful in menstruation and the water gained at this time. It is excellent for insomnia.

B-12: This nutrient increases the body's resistance to infection. A person especially needs this vitamin when fatigued. It helps form red blood cells, and helps prevent constipation.

BIOTIN: It is used for the proper functioning of skin, nerves, bone marrow, and reproductive glands. It helps metabolize carbohydrates and protein.

CHOLINE: This vitamin helps keep the nerve coverings (myelin) healthy, and aids in production of acetycholine, (a neurotransmitter), and helps the body utilize fat and cholesterol.

FOLIC ACID: It is used for red blood cell formation and the synthesis of inositol. It works with choline and is vital for nourishment of the brain. It has been shown to help reduce fat in the liver.

PABA (Para-Aminobenzoic Acid): This vitamin protects the body against free radicals and is part of the folic acid molecule.

FOOD SOURCES OF IMMUNE BUILDERS

Minerals

CALCIUM: Milk and milk products, all cheeses, soybeans, sardines, salmon, peanuts, walnuts, sunflower seeds, dried beans, green vegetables.

CHROMIUM: Meat, shellfish, chicken, corn oil, clams, brewer's yeast.

IODINE: Kelp, vegetables grown in iodine-rich soil, onions, and all seafood.

MAGNESIUM: Figs, lemons, grapefruit, yellow corn, almonds, nuts, seeds, dark green vegetables, apples.

MANGANESE: Nuts, green leafy vegetables, peas, beets, eggs, egg yolks, whole wheat cereals.

SELENIUM: Wheat germ, bran, tuna, onions, tomatoes, broccoli.

ZINC: Round steak, lamb chops, pork loin, wheat germ, brewer's yeast, pumpkin seeds, eggs, nonfat dry milk, ground mustard.

Vitamins

VITAMIN A: Orange and bright green fruits and vegetables, peppers, peaches, apricots, cod liver oil, carrots, yams.

VITAMIN E: Wheat germ, nuts, sweet potatoes, corn, sunflower oil, spinach, watercress, tomatoes

VITAMIN C: Most fruits and vegetables, especially citrus fruits and green peppers.

B-1: Whole grain wheat, whole grain oats, lentils, navy beans, pinto beans, red beans, and many vegetables.

B-2: Mushrooms, millet, split peas, barley, parsley, broccoli, chicken, turkey, lentils, many beans, okra and almonds.

B-3: Turkey, chicken, brown rice, buckwheat, mushrooms, barley, red chili peppers, split peas, dates, and brewer's yeast.

B-5: Foods include whole grains, green vegetables, nuts, meats and fish.

B-6: Cantaloupe, tuna, lentils, buckwheat, whole grain rice, bananas, whole grain rye, spinach, potatoes, and many other fruits and vegetables.

B-12: Liver, milk, eggs, meat, cheese, miso, and soy sauce.

19

BIOTIN: Peas, peanuts, beans, lentils, milk, whole grain rice, beef liver, fish, and whole grains.
CHOLINE: Lecithin, leafy green vegetables, oats, soybeans, egg yolks, and liver.
FOLIC ACID: Fresh dark green vegetables, carrots, cantaloupes, apricots, beans, whole wheat flour, endive, asparagus and turnips.
INOSITOL: Cabbage, grapefruit, cantaloupe, peanuts, raisins, lima beans.

Since AIDS sufferers are usually always afflicted with the fungus Candida Albicans, they are advised to avoid foods which will feed this yeast infestation. The following are lists of "Foods to Avoid" and "Foods to Enjoy", and "Use Occasionally".

Foods to Avoid:
All sugar products, maple syrup, honey, and any sweeteners; dairy products, except butter; bread and pastries; alcoholic beverages; mushrooms and all fungi, molds and yeast in any form. All pickled products: salad dressings, green olives, relishes, and pickled relishes. All fermented foods: sauerkraut, soy sauce, tamari. All dry roasted nuts. Avoid potato chips, pretzels, crackers. Avoid soda pop, white flour products, bacon, salt pork, lunch meats and cheese of all kinds. Avoid leftover food, where molds and yeast grow and thrive.

Foods to Enjoy:
Eggs, fish, chicken, turkey, lamb and/or veal. Organically fed animals that are not injected with antibiotics and hormones. All vegetables, except potatoes (occasionally), corn and yams. Onions, garlic, cabbage, broccoli, turnips, brussel sprouts, kohlrabi and winter squash. Kelp and paprika for seasoning, along with lemon and cold-pressed oils. Stews, using vegetables, tomatoes, chicken and lamb. Millet, brown rice, buckwheat, and wild rice dishes, small amounts at first. Use millet or rice cakes instead of bread. Muffins and cornbreads are okay. Avocado, use in salads or stuffed.
Use Occasionally:
Some whole grains, baked potatoes, fruits in small amounts, raw nuts and seeds in small amounts, dry beans and legumes (small amounts), millet, brown rice, buckwheat and yellow cornmeal.

HOW TO PREVENT AIDS

A strong immune system is the key to avoiding any disease. Since AIDS is primarily transmitted through homosexual activities, the best prevention is to avoid the type of behavior that transmits the AIDS virus. Homosexual acts go against the way and reasons nature designed us as human beings. Promiscuous behavior in any form will reap the consequences. Old-fashioned virtue is still the best bet at any price.

OTHER IMMUNE SYSTEM STRENGTHENERS:

EXERCISE: Exercising for at least fifteen minutes a day will elevate the white blood cell count in your body. The white blood cells are the germ-fighters of the immune system. Exercise helps stimulate lymphatic flow and blood circulation, thus promoting oxygen to the brain and all areas of the body. It helps minimize stress and its detrimental effects.

POSITIVE MENTAL ATTITUDE: Studies and research prove that a positive state of mind boosts the body's immunity by releasing infection-fighting T-cells from the thymus gland.

RAW FOOD DIET: The importance of correct diet in relation to the immune system cannot be overemphasized. Cooked, preservative-loaded, synthetic-additive food is dead--it has no life. If it has no life, it has no ability to sustain life. The body's cells will deteriorate without proper nutrition to vitalize them. Raw fruits and vegetables, and also the fresh juices made from them, will provide necessary enzymes, vitamins and minerals that the body needs. This in turn, will aid the immune system in combatting toxins, bacteria, molds and fungi. Whole grains supply B-vitamins, which are necessary for both the nervous and immune systems. It is best not to cook the grains with high heat, but let them soak in a thermos overnight with boiling water poured over the grain. This is known as "the thermos method". Taheebo (Pau d'Arco) Tea is very, very beneficial to combat viruses and strengthen the immune system. Drink several times daily.

MENUS AND RECIPES
(The recipes marked with an * are from "Today's Healthy Eating"
by Louise Tenney, and are found in the back of this book.)

Seven Day Suggested Menu

#1 Breakfast
Cracked wheat mush with almond milk

#1 Lunch
Garden Salad*
1 piece cornbread

#1 Supper
Millet Nut Loaf*
1 cup baked beans
Steamed carrot slices
Taheebo Tea

#2 Breakfast
1 cup Buckwheat Groats* with nut milk
1/4 cup raw almonds

#2 Lunch
1 chicken breast, baked, sprinkled with lemon juice and herbs
1 cup steamed broccoli with sesame seeds
Taheebo Tea

#2 Supper
Vegetable Broth #1
Baked fish with lemon and butter
Taheebo Tea

#3 Breakfast
Brown rice, cooked with cashew milk
Poached egg

#3 Lunch
Parsley Cucumber Salad*

22

1 piece cornbread
Taheebo Tea

#3 Supper
Spring Salad
Taheebo Tea

#4 Breakfast
Cooked rice
Scrambled egg with sweet basil herbs and green onions

#4 Lunch
Raw Soup #1*
10 raw almonds
Taheebo Tea

#4 Supper
Baked Rice and Millet*
Steamed green beans
Taheebo Tea

#5 Breakfast
Baked yam mashed, with cinnamon
(delicious served cold, cook night before)

#5 Lunch
Avocado, sliced, sprinkled with vegetable seasoning and lemon
juice
Fresh sliced tomato
10 almonds
Taheebo Tea

#5 Supper
Yogurt Gazpacho*
Carrot sticks
Taheebo Tea

#6 Breakfast
Thermos Millet*

AIDS

<u>#6 Lunch</u>
Raw Soup #2*
Celery sticks
Taheebo Tea

<u>#6 Supper</u>
Steamed combo of brussels sprouts, tomatoes, and onions, with
  Italian herb seasoning. Serve over rice with tomato sauce
Taheebo Tea

<u>#7 Breakfast</u>
Cooked millet with cashew milk

<u>#7 Lunch</u>
Beet Salad*, sprinkled with raw sunflower seeds
Steamed carrots, mashed with butter

<u>#7 Dinner</u>
Baked potato with plain yogurt, lemon juice, chopped green on-
ions (green part)
Bean soup

RECIPES

<u>Nut Milks:</u>

ALMOND MILK

1 C. almonds, ground
1 quart pure water
2 T. pure maple syrup (optional)

Blend thoroughly in a blender until it is smooth. Strain through a
strainer or cheese cloth.

SESAME MILK

1 C. sesame seeds
1 quart pure water
2 T. pure maple syrup (optional)

Blend ingredients in a blender until smooth and strain off the milk.

COCONUT MILK

1 1/2 C. grated fresh coconut
1 quart pure water
2 T. sunflower oil

Blend all together and strain off milk.

NUT AND SEED MILK

1/2 C. blanched almonds
1/2 C. sesame seeds
1 quart pure water
2 T. pure maple syrup

Blend together in blender and strain the milk.

GARDEN SALAD

3 C. leaf lettuce
1/2 C. fresh peas, shelled
1/2 C. carrots, grated
1/2 C. zuchini, grated

1 cucumber
1/2 avocado
1/2 C. mixed sunflower seeds and ground almonds

Mix all ingredients together. Serve with lemon juice or herb dressing.

MILLET NUT LOAF

2 C. cooked millet	1 medium onion
1 C. walnuts, almonds, pecans ground fine	1 egg
	1/4 C. red pepper
2 tsp. vegetable seasoning broth	4 medium ripe tomatoes

Blend together and bake in oven at 350°F for one hour. Serve with tomato sauce.

BUCKWHEAT GROATS

2 C. buckwheat groats	1 tsp. vegetable salt
2 eggs, lightly beaten	4 C. pure water, boiled

Cook groats and eggs in a heavy skillet over a high heat for a few minutes. Stir constantly to keep eggs from sticking. Add boiling water and reduce heat and simmer, covered, for about 30 minutes. Add vegetable salt before serving.

VEGETABLE BROTH #1

1 gallon pure water	6 medium potatoes, scrubbed with skins on
2 large onions	
2 leeks	4 medium carrots
1 C. fresh parsley	1 bay leaf
2 parsnips	1/2 tsp. thyme
2 turnips	1/2 tsp. basil
4 ribs celery	1/2 tsp. rosemary
1 medium green pepper	1 T. vegetable seasoning

Combine all ingredients in a large stainless steel pan with the gallon of water. Bring to boil, lower heat and simmer for about 1-1/2 hours. Strain and use for soups and stews.

PARSLEY-CUCUMBER SALAD

1/2 C. parsley	1 C. cucumbers, sliced
1/2 C. sweet onions, sliced	2 large fresh tomatoes, chopped

Dressing:

1/2 C. feta cheese	1/4 tsp. oregano
1/4 C. Sunflower seed oil	1/2 C. sesame seeds ground
2 T. lemon juice	
1 clove garlic, ground	1 tsp. paprika
Dash white pepper	

SPRING SALAD

1 C. watercress	1/4 C. Jerusalem arti-
1 C. dandelion greens	chokes grated
1 small red onion	Bunch parsley leaves

Wash greens and pat dry. Tear into small pieces. Grate artichokes into salad. Chop onion, add greens, and serve with oil and lemon juice dressing.

RAW SOUP #1

Raw soups contain live enzymes that are essential to help the immune system.

3 C. vegetable broth	1 T. olive oil
1 C. tomato juice	1/2 tsp. kelp
1 T. ground chia seeds	2 T. vegetable broth powder

Heat all ingredients and simmer for 10 minutes. Remove from heat and add the following raw vegetables:

1/2 C. grated carrots	1 small chopped onion
1/2 C. grated celery	2 fresh tomatoes cut in small pieces
1/2 C. fresh sweet corn	
1/2 C. fresh peas	2 sprigs parsley, chopped

AIDS

BAKED RICE AND MILLET

1-1/2 C. cooked brown
   rice
1/2 C. cooked millet
2 eggs, beaten
2 C. milk

2 T. butter
1 T. tamari soy sauce
1 C. chopped almonds
1/4 C. chopped sunflower
   seeds

Mix all ingredients. Pour into 1 1/2 quart casserole dish. Bake 30 minutes at 350°F.

YOGURT GAzPACHO

1 1/2 C. yogurt
4-1/2 T. olive oil
2 cloves garlic
1 green pepper
4 tomatoes, peeled and
   chopped

1 medium cucumber,
   peeled and chopped
1/2 tsp. basil
1/2 tsp. cumin
2 T. cider vinegar

Mix in a blender all the ingredients and chill well before serving.

RAW SOUP #2

4 C. pure water
1 C. small cubed
   potatoes, skin on
1 clove garlic

1 medium onion
2 T. vegetable broth powder

Simmer all ingredients together until potatoes are done. Remove from stove and add the following ingredients.

1 C. grated carrots
1/2 C. chopped celery
1/2 C. finely chopped green
   beans

1/2 C. chopped spinach
1/2 C. chopped parsley

Serve immediately for a live enzyme soup.

BEET SALAD

2 C. red cabbage, shredded 1 C. parsnips, grated
1 C. beets, grated, raw 1 C. watercress
1 C. carrots, grated 2 T. parsley, minced

Arrange the shredded cabbage on a platter. Stir French dressing separately with carrots, parsnips and beets, and place them separately on the cabbage bed. Sprinkle parsley and watercress on the top.

BEAN SOUP

1 C. navy beans 1/2 C. parsley, chopped
4 C. pure water 1 T. nut cream
1 C. grated carrots 1 tsp. lemon juice
1 small onion, grated

Soak beans overnight in three cups of water. Cook beans in 4 cups water until tender. Blend the cooked beans and vegetables in a blender, add parsley, nut cream and lemon and let boil for a few minutes. Ready to serve.

RECOMMENDED READING

Aids Cover-up, by Gene Antonio.
Candida Albicans: A Nutritional Approach, by Louise Tenney
Today's Healthy Eating, by Louise Tenney.